INTERMITTENT

FASTING

FOR WOMEN

OVER 50

SARAH JACK

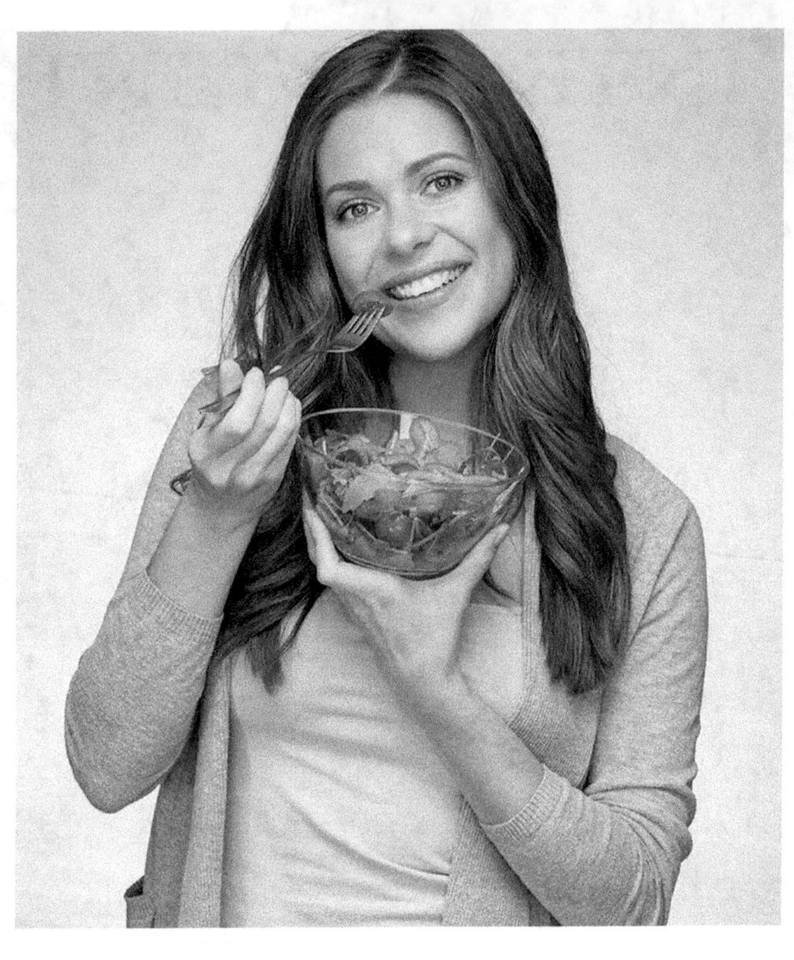

COPYRIGHT

All rights reserved. This book or any portion thereof may not be reproduced or used in any manner whatsoever without the express written permission of the publisher except for the use of brief quotations in a book review.

TABLE OF CONTENTS

INTRODUCTION

The eating pattern known as intermittent fasting (IF) alternates between periods of fasting and eating. The idea of fasting for health or religious reasons has been practiced for centuries across many countries, though it has seen a substantial increase in popularity in recent years. An outline of the background of intermittent fasting is provided below:

- **Ancient Times:** Fasting has a long history and has been used by many cultures for religious and spiritual objectives. For instance, several major religions, including Christianity, Islam, and Judaism, practice fasting regularly. Fasting was frequently linked to atonement, self-control, and communion with the divine.

- **Early Medical Interest:** Intermittent fasting attracted medical interest in the early 20th century. Researchers have studied fasting and its potential health benefits, including Dr. Benjamin Horace Phinney. Although its efficacy varied, fasting was occasionally utilized as a treatment for obesity and other medical disorders.

- **1950s–1960s:** As pharmaceutical treatments and calorie-restricted diets gained popularity, interest in fasting dwindled. Fasting's popularity decreased in favor of alternative weight loss techniques since it was perceived as excessive and potentially hazardous.

- **1980s–2000s:** Animal studies and sporadic human studies persisted in investigating the potential health advantages of intermittent fasting. Time-restricted feeding and alternate-day fasting were ideas that attracted some interest, but they were not extensively used.

- **Early in the twenty-first century:** In the 2000s, both scholarly and lay circles once again paid attention to intermittent fasting. IF entered the mainstream in 2013 with the release of studies and publications like "The Fast Diet" by Michael Mosley and Mimi Spencer. The 5:2 diet, in which people eat normally for five days and follow an extremely low-calorie diet for the other two, gained popularity thanks to this **book.**

- **Recent Popularity:** Due to its potential advantages for weight management, metabolic health, and lifespan, intermittent fasting has grown significantly in popularity over the past ten years. Many people now recognize and use variations of intermittent fasting, such as the 16/8 approach (fasting for 16 hours and eating within an 8-hour window) and the 12/12 method.

- **Scientific Research:** Yoshinori Ohsumi received the 2016 Nobel Prize in Physiology or Medicine for his studies on the mechanics of autophagy, a cellular process that takes place when a person fasts and has ramifications for their health and longevity. This understanding stoked even more interest in intermittent fasting and its conceivable health advantages.

- Studies are still being conducted to determine how intermittent fasting affects a variety of health indicators, such as insulin sensitivity, weight loss, brain function, and more. The scientific community is currently actively looking into the long-term consequences and best practices for various populations as of my most recent update in September 2021.

Finally, it should be noted that while intermittent fasting has long been a part of religious and cultural traditions, its modern resurgence may be dated to the first decade of the twenty-first century. A combination of academic studies, publications, and individual success stories have increased its appeal. Individual responses to intermittent fasting, it should be noted, can vary, therefore it is advised to speak with a healthcare provider before making any significant dietary adjustments.

INTERMITTENT FASTING

Intermittent fasting, a nutritional phenomenon gaining increasing attention, has emerged as a transformative approach to eating for various health benefits. This dietary strategy revolves around alternating periods of eating and fasting, harnessing the body's natural processes to promote overall well-being. In this exploration, we delve into the science, methods, benefits, challenges, and practical aspects of intermittent fasting.

- **UNDERSTANDING THE BASICS**

➢ Definition and Principles:

Intermittent fasting involves cycling between periods of eating and fasting. Rather than focusing on what to eat, it places emphasis on when to eat. The fundamental principle is to create intentional periods of food deprivation, allowing the body to utilize stored energy efficiently.

➢ **Mechanism Behind Intermittent Fasting:**

During fasting periods, the body shifts from using glucose as its primary energy source to burning stored fat. This metabolic transition triggers various cellular repair processes and activates autophagy, a cellular cleansing mechanism. Additionally, fasting is known to influence hormone levels, including insulin and human growth hormone, contributing to improved metabolic health.

- **METHODS OF INTERMITTENT FASTING**

➢ **The 16/8 Method:**

One of the most popular approaches, the 16/8 method, involves daily fasting for 16 hours and restricting eating to an 8-hour window. This method is practical for many individuals as it can be easily incorporated into daily routines.

➢ **The 5:2 Diet:**

In the 5:2 diet, individuals consume a regular diet for five days a week and limit calorie intake to around 500-600 calories on two non-consecutive fasting days. This method offers flexibility, allowing for normal eating on non-fasting days.

➢ **Alternate-Day Fasting:**

As the name suggests, alternate-day fasting involves alternating between days of regular eating and days of either complete fasting or significant calorie reduction. While it can be effective, it may pose challenges in adherence for some individuals.

➢ **Extended Fasting:**

Extended fasting typically involves fasting for periods longer than 24 hours, ranging from 48 hours to several days. This method requires careful consideration and supervision due to the extended duration of food deprivation.

- **THE BENEFITS OF INTERMITTENT FASTING**

➢ **Weight Management:**

Intermittent fasting has gained popularity for its potential to aid weight loss. By creating a calorie deficit during fasting periods, the body relies on stored fat for energy, contributing to fat loss. Moreover, the metabolic effects of fasting may enhance weight loss compared to traditional calorie-restricted diets.

➢ **Improved Metabolic Health:**

Studies indicate that intermittent fasting can positively impact metabolic health by reducing insulin resistance and promoting better blood sugar control. These effects are particularly relevant for individuals at risk of type 2 diabetes.

➢ **Cognitive Benefits:**

Fasting has been associated with cognitive benefits, including improved brain function and protection against age-related neurodegenerative diseases. The increased production of brain-derived neurotrophic factor (BDNF) during fasting supports cognitive health.

➢ **Longevity and Aging:**

Research in animals suggests that intermittent fasting may extend lifespan and improve overall longevity. While the evidence in humans is still evolving, the cellular repair mechanisms activated during fasting are believed to contribute to the anti-aging effects.

➢ **Cellular Repair Processes:**

Autophagy, a process where cells remove damaged components, is upregulated during fasting. This cellular cleansing mechanism is essential for maintaining cellular health and preventing the accumulation of dysfunctional components.

- **ADDRESSING CHALLENGES AND CONCERNS**

➤ **Hunger and Satiety:**

One of the primary challenges of intermittent fasting is dealing with hunger during fasting periods. However, many individuals report adapting to this over time, and staying adequately hydrated can help manage hunger.

➤ **Social and Lifestyle Considerations:**

Social situations, family meals, and cultural practices can pose challenges to adhering to a fasting regimen. Flexible approaches, such as adjusting fasting windows, can help integrate fasting into diverse lifestyles.

➤ **Potential Nutrient Deficiencies:**

Long-term adherence to specific fasting methods may lead to nutrient deficiencies. It is crucial to prioritize nutrient-dense foods and consider supplementation when necessary.

- **GETTING STARTED AND STAYING CONSISTENT**

➤ **Consultation with Healthcare Professionals:**

Before embarking on an intermittent fasting journey, it is advisable to consult with healthcare professionals, especially for individuals with existing health conditions or those taking medications.

➤ **Choosing the Right Fasting Method:**

Selecting a fasting method that aligns with individual preferences, lifestyle, and health goals is essential. The flexibility of intermittent fasting allows individuals to experiment and find the approach that suits them best.

➤ **Setting Realistic Goals:**

Establishing realistic and achievable goals is fundamental to long-term success. Whether the aim is weight loss, improved metabolic health, or enhanced cognitive function, setting incremental goals contributes to sustained motivation.

➢ **Monitoring Progress:**

Tracking key metrics, such as weight, energy levels, and overall well-being, helps individuals assess the impact of intermittent fasting on their health. Adjustments can be made based on individual responses.

- **THE ROLE OF EXERCISE IN INTERMITTENT FASTING**

Exercise complements intermittent fasting, contributing to overall health and well-being. Engaging in regular physical activity supports metabolic health, enhances fat loss, and promotes cardiovascular fitness. Combining appropriate exercise routines with intermittent fasting can amplify the benefits of both.

- **FINAL THOUGHTS**

Intermittent fasting is a dynamic and evolving field of research that has shown promising results in various aspects of health and wellness. While it may not be suitable for everyone, many individuals find it to be a sustainable and effective approach to improve their overall health.

As with any lifestyle change, it is essential to approach intermittent fasting with awareness, mindfulness, and a commitment to individualized well-being. Consulting with healthcare professionals, staying informed about the latest research, and listening to one's body are integral components of a successful intermittent fasting journey. Ultimately, intermittent fasting is not just about changing when we eat but about embracing a holistic approach to health and vitality.

WOMEN OVER 50

Entering the age of 50 marks a significant milestone for women, and it often comes with both challenges and opportunities. This stage of life is characterized by unique physiological changes, evolving priorities, and a continued pursuit of well-being. In this comprehensive guide, we explore the multifaceted aspects of women's health over 50, covering physical health, mental well-being, lifestyle considerations, and strategies for embracing this vibrant phase of life.

- **PHYSICAL HEALTH**

➢ **Hormonal Changes:**

As women enter their 50s, hormonal shifts, particularly related to menopause, become a focal point. Understanding and managing these changes are crucial for maintaining overall health. Regular health check-ups and consultations with healthcare professionals can help navigate this transition, addressing concerns such as hot flashes, hormonal imbalances, and bone health.

➢ Bone Health:

Osteoporosis becomes a more significant consideration for women over 50. Adequate calcium and vitamin D intake, along with weight-bearing exercises, are vital for maintaining bone density. Bone density scans and discussions with healthcare providers can guide preventive measures.

➢ Heart Health:

Cardiovascular health gains prominence, and women in their 50s should focus on maintaining healthy cholesterol levels, blood pressure, and heart function. Regular exercise, a heart-healthy diet, and stress management contribute to cardiovascular well-being.

➢ **Weight Management:**

Metabolism tends to slow down with age, making weight management more challenging. Embracing a balanced diet rich in nutrients and engaging in regular physical activity are fundamental. Women over 50 may find that a combination of strength training and aerobic exercise is particularly beneficial.

➢ Regular Health Screenings:

Regular health screenings become even more critical in the 50s. Mammograms, Pap smears, colonoscopies, and other age-appropriate screenings aid in early detection and prevention of various health conditions.

- **MENTAL WELL-BEING**

➢ **Cognitive Health:**

Cognitive well-being becomes a focus in the 50s. Engaging in activities that stimulate the mind, such as puzzles, reading, and learning new skills, can contribute to cognitive health.

Additionally, staying socially connected and maintaining an active lifestyle supports mental agility.

➢ **Stress Management:**

The 50s often bring a combination of personal and professional responsibilities. Stress management techniques, including mindfulness, meditation, and hobbies, play a crucial role in promoting mental resilience. Prioritizing self-care becomes a cornerstone of well-being.

➢ **Sleep Quality:**

Quality sleep becomes increasingly important for overall health. Establishing a consistent sleep routine, creating a comfortable sleep environment, and addressing any sleep disturbances contribute to restful nights.

➢ **Embracing Change:**

The 50s can be a period of significant life changes, including career transitions, empty nesting, or even becoming a grandparent. Embracing these changes with a positive mindset, seeking support when needed, and focusing on personal growth contribute to a fulfilling life.

- **LIFESTYLE CONSIDERATIONS**

➢ **Nutrition:**

Nutrient-dense, balanced eating is crucial for women over 50. Adequate protein, calcium, and vitamins are essential. Consulting with a nutritionist can help tailor dietary choices to individual needs and address any specific health concerns.

➢ **Physical Activity:**

Regular exercise remains a cornerstone of well-being. Incorporating a mix of aerobic activities, strength training, and flexibility exercises supports overall fitness. Women over 50 should choose activities they enjoy to promote adherence.

➢ **Social Connections:**

Maintaining social connections is paramount for emotional well-being. Joining clubs, participating in community events, or staying connected with friends and family helps combat feelings of isolation.

➢ **Hobbies and Passions:**

Pursuing hobbies and passions becomes a source of joy and fulfillment. Whether it's art, gardening, travel, or learning a musical instrument, dedicating time to personal interests contributes to a well-rounded and satisfying life.

➢ **Financial Planning:**

The 50s are a critical time for financial planning. Evaluating retirement goals, managing investments, and ensuring financial security are essential considerations. Seeking advice from financial professionals can provide guidance in navigating this aspect of life.

- **STRATEGIES FOR EMBRACING LIFE IN THE 50S**

➢ **Mindful Aging:**

Embracing the aging process with mindfulness and a positive outlook is transformative. Accepting the changes that come with age while celebrating achievements and experiences contributes to a sense of fulfillment.

➢ **Regular Check-Ups:**

Regular health check-ups, including eye exams, dental visits, and screenings for various health conditions, are proactive measures for overall well-being. Staying informed about one's health status allows for timely interventions when needed.

➢ **Continued Learning:**

The 50s are an excellent time for continued learning and personal development. Whether pursuing formal education, attending workshops, or exploring new interests, the quest for **knowledge remains invigorating.**

➢ **Cultivating Gratitude:**

Cultivating a sense of gratitude for life's blessings, both big and small, fosters a positive mindset. Keeping a gratitude journal or regularly reflecting on positive aspects of life contributes to emotional well-being.

➢ **Community Involvement:**

Active involvement in the community, through volunteering or participating in local initiatives, provides a sense of purpose and connection. Contributing to causes that align with personal values adds meaning to daily life.

• **CONCLUSION**

Navigating the journey of being a woman over 50 involves a holistic approach to well-being—addressing physical health, nurturing mental resilience, embracing lifestyle choices, and adopting strategies that enhance the quality of life. With a focus on proactive health measures, a positive mindset, and a commitment to personal growth, women in their 50s can continue to lead vibrant, fulfilling lives. As every woman's journey is unique, it's essential to tailor these strategies to individual preferences, needs, and aspirations, creating a roadmap for a flourishing and ageless future.

BENEFITS OF INTERMITTENT FASTING FOR WOMEN OVER 50

Women over 50 may benefit from intermittent fasting (IF), but it's crucial to approach the practice with an awareness of the distinct physiological changes brought on by advancing age. For women in this age range, intermittent fasting may have the following advantages:

- Weight management might be difficult as we age since our metabolisms tend to slow down. A calorie deficit is necessary for weight loss or weight maintenance and can be produced with the use of IF. Lean muscle mass preservation during weight loss is another benefit.

- Improved Insulin Sensitivity: Type 2 diabetes risk can be raised by aging, which is frequently correlated with lower insulin sensitivity. IF could increase insulin sensitivity, assisting in controlling blood sugar levels and lowering the chance of developing diabetes.

- Cardiovascular Health: IF may result in better blood pressure, cholesterol, and inflammatory levels, which are all indicators of cardiovascular health. These advantages may help reduce the risk of heart disease.

- Improved brain health and cognitive performance have been associated with IF. It might promote the development of new neurons, offer defense against neurodegenerative conditions, and improve concentration and memory.

- Bone Health: Postmenopausal women, who are more likely to develop osteoporosis, need to consume enough nutrients to maintain healthy bones. It is important to follow IF in a way that assures enough consumption of calcium, vitamin D, and other minerals that maintain healthy bones.

- Hormone Regulation: The menopause can cause hormonal changes that affect the body's metabolism and composition. According to some research, IF may help control the hormones responsible for controlling appetite and controlling weight.

- Cellular Repair and Longevity: IF starts the cellular repair process known as autophagy, which eliminates harmed cells and cellular parts. This procedure is believed to contribute to lifetime extension and better aging.

- Sustainable Lifestyle: Due to its simplicity compared to sophisticated food plans, IF may be simpler for some women over 50 to adhere to. This can make it a more long-term strategy for keeping up a healthy weight and way of life.

- Joint Health: IF may result in less inflammation, which is good for joints and may help treat diseases like arthritis.

- Eating within a constrained time frame helps improve nutritional absorption and utilization, ensuring that the body gets the most out of the nutrients taken.

- Benefits for the Mind: Some women claim that fasting improves their mood, mental clarity, and ability to concentrate. This could have a favorable effect on their general health.

- Empowerment and Body Confidence: Adopting intermittent fasting successfully can promote a feeling of empowerment and body confidence, which helps to boost one's self-esteem.

Despite these possible advantages, it's crucial to understand that everyone will react to intermittent fasting differently. Some fasting patterns may be more suited to women than others. Particularly for women over 50, it is advised to speak with a healthcare provider before beginning an intermittent fasting regimen to make sure that any pre-existing medical concerns or dietary requirements are taken into account.

Gaining the benefits of intermittent fasting requires a

consistent and balanced approach.

POTENTIAL RISKS AND SIDE EFFECTS OF INTERMITTENT FASTING

Intermittent fasting has garnered attention for its potential benefits, from weight management to improved metabolic health. However, like any dietary approach, it is essential to examine potential risks and side effects associated with this fasting pattern. While intermittent fasting is generally considered safe for many individuals, it is crucial to understand that its impact can vary based on factors such as individual health, existing medical conditions, and adherence to proper guidelines.

- **Potential Risks and Side Effects:**

Nutrient Deficiency:

Intermittent fasting may lead to nutrient deficiencies if not carefully planned. Inadequate nutrient intake during eating windows could impact overall health and well-being. It is crucial to prioritize nutrient-dense foods when breaking a fast.

Disordered Eating Patterns:

For some individuals, intermittent fasting may contribute to disordered eating patterns. The structured nature of fasting may trigger unhealthy relationships with food or exacerbate existing issues, especially in those with a history of eating disorders.

Impact on Women's Health:

Women, particularly those in the reproductive age group, may be more susceptible to hormonal imbalances with intermittent fasting. Irregular menstrual cycles and disruptions to reproductive health have been reported in some cases.

Hypoglycemia:

Individuals prone to low blood sugar levels (hypoglycemia) should approach intermittent fasting cautiously. Extended fasting periods may lead to fluctuations in blood sugar levels, resulting in symptoms such as dizziness, fatigue, or irritability.

Difficulty Sustaining Long-Term:

Intermittent fasting may be challenging to sustain over the long term for some individuals. The rigid eating patterns may not align with everyone's lifestyle, potentially leading to inconsistent adherence.

Potential Impact on Physical Performance:

Athletes or highly active individuals may experience decreased performance during fasting periods. Adequate nutrient intake around workouts is crucial for optimal energy levels and recovery.

Sleep Disturbances:

Some individuals may experience sleep disturbances, particularly if fasting periods coincide with nighttime. Disruptions to circadian rhythms may impact sleep quality.

Gastrointestinal Issues:

Extended fasting periods may lead to gastrointestinal issues such as bloating, constipation, or acid reflux. The absence of regular meals can affect the digestive system.

Impact on Mental Health:

While intermittent fasting is not inherently linked to mental health issues, some individuals may experience increased irritability, mood swings, or heightened stress levels during fasting periods.

Social Challenges:

Adopting intermittent fasting may present challenges in social settings where meals are a central aspect of social interaction. Fasting periods may conflict with social norms and activities.

- **Individualized Approach and Mitigation Strategies:**

Consultation with Healthcare Professionals:

Before embarking on intermittent fasting, especially for those with existing health conditions, consulting healthcare professionals is crucial. They can provide personalized guidance based on individual health needs.

Mindful Eating:

Practicing mindful eating during non-fasting periods helps ensure that individuals consume a balanced and nutrient-dense diet. Emphasis should be placed on whole foods to meet nutritional requirements.

Hydration:

Staying adequately hydrated is essential during fasting periods. Water, herbal teas, and other non-caloric beverages can help maintain hydration levels.

Gradual Adaptation:

For individuals new to intermittent fasting, a gradual adaptation approach can be beneficial. Starting with shorter fasting periods and progressively extending them allows the body to adjust.

Monitoring for Adverse Effects:

Regular monitoring of individual responses is crucial. If adverse effects, such as fatigue, dizziness, or mood changes, are experienced, adjustments to the fasting approach may be necessary.

Consideration for Women's Health:

Women, especially those in reproductive age groups, should be attentive to potential hormonal impacts. Consulting with healthcare providers can help tailor fasting strategies to individual needs.

Strategic Planning for Athletes:

Athletes or those with high physical activity levels should strategically plan nutrient intake around workouts to support energy needs and recovery.

Conclusion: A Balanced Perspective on Intermittent Fasting:

Intermittent fasting offers a unique approach to eating that has shown promise in various studies. However, it is not a one-size-fits-all solution, and potential risks and side effects should be carefully considered. Adopting an individualized and mindful approach, consulting healthcare professionals, and staying attuned to the body's responses can contribute to a balanced perspective on intermittent fasting.

As with any dietary approach, what works for one person may not be suitable for another. Striking a balance between reaping potential benefits and mitigating risks ensures a holistic and sustainable approach to intermittent fasting. The key lies in informed decision-making, personalized strategies, and a focus on overall well-being.

DIETARY PLANS FOR INTERMITTENT FASTING METHODS

Finding a balanced strategy to satisfy nutritional requirements while taking into account the possible advantages of fasting is important when developing an intermittent fasting (IF) diet plan for women over 50. Here is a sample diet that you may use as a jumping off point. However, keep in mind that everyone has different needs and preferences, so it's crucial to adapt this plan to your particular situation and speak with a healthcare professional before making any major dietary adjustments.

- **The 16/8 Method (16 hours of fasting followed by an 8-hour interval for eating)**

Eating Hours: 12 PM to 8 PM

➢ Lunch will be grilled chicken salad with mixed greens, cherry tomatoes, cucumbers, avocado, and vinaigrette dressing at 12:00 PM.

➢ Greek yogurt, a large handful of almonds, and a dash of cinnamon for a snack at three o'clock.

➢ Dinner will be salmon baked with quinoa and roasted veggies, such as broccoli, carrots, and bell peppers, at 6:00 PM.

➢ A piece of fruit, such as an apple or a small bowl of berries, for dessert at 7:30 p.m.

- **The 5:2 Method (two days of 500–600 calorie fasting followed by five days of regular eating):**

Days of Fasting: 500–600 calories

➢ Breakfast would consist of a tiny piece of whole-grain toast and scrambled eggs with spinach.

➤ Lunch will be a quinoa salad with grilled vegetables and a simple vinaigrette.

➤ Dinner will consist of baked chicken breast, steamed broccoli, and a tiny amount of brown rice.

● **Use the Eat-Stop-Eat Method (a 24-hour fast once or twice each week):**

Day of Fasting:

➤ Drink water and herbal tea in the morning to stay hydrated.

➤ Lunch will consist of a salad and a broth-based vegetable soup.

➤ Dinner will be a sizable salad with a variety of veggies, grilled tofu, and a mild dressing.

- **Alternate-Day Fasting: This involves fasting every other day.**

Day of Fasting:

➢ Black coffee or herbal tea in the morning.

➢ Lunch will be a stir-fry of vegetables and chickpeas with a modest amount of brown rice.

➢ Hummus and carrot and cucumber sticks for a snack.

➢ Dinner will consist of lentil soup and steamed asparagus.

- **Warrior Diet (a 20-hour fast followed by a 4-hour window for eating at night):**

Eating Hours: 6:00 PM – 10:00 PM

➢ Small Meal): Quinoa salad with diced grilled chicken, chopped vegetables, and a light vinaigrette around 6:00 PM.

➢ 8:00 PM (Main Course): Grilled fish, roasted sweet potatoes, and sautéed spinach on the side.

➢ Dessert is a tiny dish of Greek yogurt with some crushed almonds, honey, and a drizzle.

These model menus are created to follow the specified intermittent fasting techniques while offering a balanced diet. Always remember that choosing nutrient-dense foods, staying hydrated, and paying attention to your body's hunger and fullness cues are the keys to success with any IF strategy. It's also a good idea to modify these menus to suit your own preferences, dietary requirements, and dietary demands. Consider working with a qualified dietitian to create a customized plan if you have particular health issues or dietary requirements.

WHO SHOULD AVOID INTERMITTENT FASTING?

Intermittent fasting has gained considerable attention for its potential health benefits, ranging from weight management to improved metabolic health. However, it's essential to recognize that not everyone may benefit equally from this eating pattern. While intermittent fasting is generally considered safe for many individuals, there are specific groups who should approach it with caution or avoid it altogether.

- **CONSIDERATIONS FOR CAUTION:**

➤ **Pregnant or Breastfeeding Women:**

Pregnant and breastfeeding women have increased nutritional requirements, and any dietary changes should be made under the guidance of healthcare professionals. Intermittent fasting may not provide sufficient nutrients during critical periods of fetal development or lactation.

➢ **Individuals with a History of Eating Disorders:**

Those with a history of eating disorders, such as anorexia or bulimia, should approach intermittent fasting cautiously. The structured nature of fasting may trigger unhealthy eating behaviors or exacerbate existing issues.

➢ **Children and Adolescents:**

Growing bodies require consistent nutrient intake. Intermittent fasting may interfere with the nutritional needs of children and adolescents, potentially impacting growth and development.

➢ **Individuals with Certain Medical Conditions:**

Certain medical conditions, such as diabetes, cardiovascular diseases, or metabolic disorders, may necessitate individualized dietary approaches. Consultation with healthcare providers is crucial to ensure that fasting does not negatively impact health conditions or medication regimens.

➢ **Those Prone to Hypoglycemia:**

Individuals prone to low blood sugar levels (hypoglycemia) should exercise caution with intermittent fasting. Extended fasting periods may lead to fluctuations in blood sugar levels, potentially causing symptoms like dizziness, fatigue, or irritability.

➢ **People on Medications:**

Certain medications may require adjustments to meal timing. Those taking medications that require food intake should consult their healthcare providers before adopting intermittent fasting to avoid potential interactions or adverse effects.

➢ **Active Athletes:**

Highly active individuals, particularly athletes with intense training regimens, may require a consistent nutrient intake to support energy needs and recovery. Intermittent fasting may need careful planning to ensure optimal performance.

- **ADAPTING INTERMITTENT FASTING SAFELY:**

➢ **Gradual Transition:**

For individuals new to intermittent fasting, a gradual transition can be beneficial. Start with shorter fasting periods and progressively extend them as your body adjusts.

➢ **Listen to Your Body:**

Pay attention to hunger cues, energy levels, and overall well-being. If you experience negative symptoms, consider adjusting your fasting approach or consulting a healthcare professional.

➢ **Stay Hydrated:**

Adequate hydration is essential during fasting periods. Water, herbal teas, and other non-caloric beverages can help maintain hydration levels.

> **Balanced Nutrition:**

Focus on nutrient-dense foods during eating windows to ensure that your body receives essential vitamins and minerals. Emphasize a balanced diet rich in whole foods.

> **Consultation with Professionals:**

Before embarking on intermittent fasting, particularly for those in high-risk groups, consulting healthcare professionals, nutritionists, or dietitians is advisable. They can provide personalized guidance based on individual health needs.

- **CONCLUSION: PERSONALIZATION IS KEY**

Intermittent fasting is not a one-size-fits-all approach, and its suitability varies based on individual factors. While many people can incorporate intermittent fasting safely into their lifestyles, certain groups need to approach it cautiously or avoid it altogether. The key is personalization—tailoring dietary choices to individual needs, health conditions, and goals.

Before adopting intermittent fasting, especially for those in vulnerable groups, seeking guidance from healthcare professionals ensures that any potential risks are mitigated, and the approach aligns with individual health requirements. As with any dietary change, a mindful and informed approach is paramount, recognizing that what works for one person may not be suitable for another. Ultimately, the goal is to foster a healthy relationship with food and prioritize overall well-being in a sustainable manner.

INTEGRATING EXERCISE AND INTERMITTENT FASTING

In the dynamic landscape of health and wellness, the synergy between exercise and intermittent fasting has emerged as a powerful combination, offering a holistic approach to achieving fitness goals and promoting overall well-being. This comprehensive guide explores the science behind both practices, their individual benefits, and the transformative effects when seamlessly integrated.

- **THE ROLE OF EXERCISE IN OVERALL HEALTH:**

➢ **Cardiovascular Benefits:**

Regular cardiovascular exercise, such as running, cycling, or brisk walking, enhances heart health by improving circulation, lowering blood pressure, and reducing the risk of cardiovascular diseases. These benefits synergize with intermittent fasting to support overall cardiovascular well-being.

➢ **Strength Training and Muscular Health:**

Engaging in strength training exercises, including weightlifting or resistance training, is crucial for maintaining muscle mass, bone density, and metabolic rate. Combining strength training with intermittent fasting promotes lean muscle preservation during fasting periods.

➢ **Flexibility and Mobility:**

Incorporating flexibility exercises, such as yoga or stretching routines, improves joint health, enhances mobility, and contributes to overall functional fitness. These activities complement the diverse range of benefits offered by intermittent fasting.

➢ **Mental Health Benefits:**

Exercise is a potent stress reliever, promoting the release of endorphins, the body's natural mood enhancers. Regular physical activity is associated with improved mental health, reduced anxiety and depression, and enhanced cognitive function—attributes that align seamlessly with the holistic approach of intermittent fasting.

- **THE SYNERGY BETWEEN EXERCISE AND INTERMITTENT FASTING:**

➢ **Enhanced Fat Utilization:**

The combination of exercise and intermittent fasting creates an environment in which the body becomes adept at utilizing stored fat for energy. Fasting periods, especially when coupled with aerobic exercise, encourage the breakdown of fatty acids, promoting fat loss.

➢ **Improved Insulin Sensitivity:**

Both exercise and intermittent fasting independently contribute to improved insulin sensitivity. When combined, they create a potent synergy in managing blood sugar levels. Exercise enhances the body's ability to uptake glucose, aligning with intermittent fasting's focus on stabilizing insulin levels.

➢ **Muscle Preservation:**

While intermittent fasting encourages the body to rely on stored fat for energy, incorporating regular strength training sessions during eating windows aids in muscle preservation. This synergistic effect is crucial for maintaining a healthy balance between fat loss and muscle mass.

➢ **Optimized Hormonal Environment:**

Exercise, particularly high-intensity interval training (HIIT), triggers the release of growth hormone and promotes muscle-building processes. When paired with intermittent fasting, these hormonal responses are further optimized, creating an environment conducive to both fat metabolism and muscle growth.

➢ **Cognitive Benefits:**

The combination of physical activity and intermittent fasting has notable cognitive benefits. Exercise increases blood flow to the brain, promoting neuroplasticity and cognitive function. Intermittent fasting, with its influence on brain-derived neurotrophic factor (BDNF), complements these effects, contributing to enhanced mental clarity and focus.

➢ **Increased Energy and Endurance:**

Regular exercise, particularly aerobic activities, enhances cardiovascular fitness, leading to increased energy levels and endurance. When strategically timed with eating windows during intermittent fasting, individuals can capitalize on sustained energy levels throughout the day.

- **PRACTICAL TIPS FOR INTEGRATION:**

➢ **Timing of Workouts:**

Consider scheduling workouts during eating windows to optimize nutrient intake for energy and recovery. For those practicing the 16/8 method, a mid-morning or early afternoon workout aligns well with the post-meal period.

➢ **Stay Hydrated:**

Proper hydration is essential, especially during fasting periods. Drink water before, during, and after exercise to stay hydrated and support overall health.

➢ **Balanced Nutrition:**

Ensure a well-balanced diet that includes sufficient protein, healthy fats, and carbohydrates to support exercise performance and recovery. Whole, nutrient-dense foods are crucial during eating windows.

➢ **Gradual Integration:**

For those new to either intermittent fasting or exercise, a gradual integration is advisable. Start with manageable durations and intensities, gradually increasing as your body adapts.

➢ **Listen to Your Body:**

Pay attention to your body's signals. If you experience fatigue, dizziness, or any discomfort, adjust your exercise intensity or consider modifying your fasting approach.

➢ **Variety in Exercise Routine:**

Incorporate a variety of exercises to engage different muscle groups and maintain overall fitness. A combination of aerobic exercise, strength training, and flexibility activities offers a well-rounded approach.

- **CONCLUSION:**

The combination of exercise and intermittent fasting embodies a synergistic approach to health that extends beyond physical fitness. By seamlessly integrating these practices, individuals can unlock a multitude of benefits—enhanced fat utilization, improved insulin sensitivity, optimized hormonal balance, and cognitive well-being. This holistic approach reflects the intricate interplay between movement and nourishment, aligning with the body's innate capacity for adaptation and optimization. As with any lifestyle change, it's crucial to consult with healthcare professionals, especially for individuals with underlying health conditions. The journey toward holistic well-being through the integration of exercise and intermittent fasting is a dynamic and personalized exploration, offering individuals the opportunity to thrive physically, mentally, and emotionally.

DELICIOUS AND NUTRIENT-PACKED RECIPES FOR INTERMITTENT FASTING

Intermittent fasting, with its focus on when to eat rather than what to eat, provides a unique approach to meal planning. Crafting delicious and nutrient-packed recipes that align with intermittent fasting principles can make the fasting windows enjoyable and satisfying. In this culinary exploration, we will delve into a variety of recipes designed to nourish the body while respecting the principles of intermittent fasting.

Avocado and Poached Egg Toast (Elevated Classic)

Ingredients:

- 1 slice whole-grain bread

- 1 ripe avocado

- 1 poached egg

- Salt and pepper to taste

- Optional toppings: cherry tomatoes, microgreens, or a drizzle of balsamic glaze

Instructions:

- Toast the whole-grain bread to your desired level of crispiness.

- Mash the ripe avocado and spread it evenly over the toasted bread.

- Place a perfectly poached egg on top of the avocado.

- Season with salt and pepper to taste.

- Garnish with cherry tomatoes, microgreens, or a drizzle of balsamic glaze for added flavor and nutrients.

Quinoa Salad with Chickpeas and Roasted Vegetables

Ingredients:

- 1 cup cooked quinoa

- 1 cup chickpeas (canned, drained, and rinsed)

- Assorted vegetables (e.g., cherry tomatoes, bell peppers, zucchini)

- Olive oil for roasting

- Fresh herbs (e.g., parsley or cilantro)

- Lemon vinaigrette (olive oil, lemon juice, Dijon mustard, salt, and pepper)

Instructions:

- Preheat the oven to 400°F (200°C).

- Toss the assorted vegetables in olive oil, salt, and pepper.

- Roast the vegetables in the oven until golden and tender.

- In a large bowl, combine cooked quinoa, chickpeas, and roasted vegetables.

- Drizzle the lemon vinaigrette over the salad and toss to combine.

- Garnish with fresh herbs for a burst of flavor.

Grilled Chicken and Vegetable Skewers

Ingredients:

- Chicken breast, cut into cubes

- Assorted vegetables (bell peppers, cherry tomatoes, red onion)

- Marinade: Olive oil, garlic, lemon juice, rosemary, salt, and pepper

Instructions:

- Prepare the marinade by combining olive oil, minced garlic, lemon juice, chopped rosemary, salt, and pepper.

- Marinate the chicken cubes in the mixture for at least 30 minutes.

- Thread the marinated chicken and assorted vegetables onto skewers.

- Grill the skewers until the chicken is cooked through and the vegetables are charred.

- Serve with a side of Greek yogurt or tzatziki for a refreshing touch.

Salmon and Asparagus Parcels

Ingredients:

- Salmon fillets

- Asparagus spears

- Lemon slices

- Fresh dill

- Olive oil, salt, and pepper

Instructions:

- Preheat the oven to 375°F (190°C).

- Place each salmon fillet on a piece of parchment paper.

- Season the salmon with olive oil, salt, and pepper.

- Arrange asparagus spears on top of the salmon fillets.

- Add lemon slices and fresh dill for added flavor.

- Fold the parchment paper to create parcels and bake until
  the salmon is cooked through.

Mediterranean Chickpea Salad

Ingredients:

- 2 cups canned chickpeas (drained and rinsed)

- Cucumber, diced

- Cherry tomatoes, halved

- Red onion, finely chopped

- Kalamata olives, sliced

- Feta cheese, crumbled

- Fresh parsley, chopped

- Dressing: Olive oil, red wine vinegar, minced garlic,
  oregano, salt, and pepper

Instructions:

- In a large bowl, combine chickpeas, diced cucumber, halved cherry tomatoes, chopped red onion, sliced Kalamata olives, crumbled feta cheese, and fresh parsley.

- In a small bowl, whisk together olive oil, red wine vinegar, minced garlic, oregano, salt, and pepper to create the dressing.

- Pour the dressing over the salad and toss to coat evenly.

- Chill the salad in the refrigerator for at least 30 minutes before serving.

Sweet Potato and Black Bean Buddha Bowl

Ingredients:

- Roasted sweet potato cubes

- Cooked black beans

- Quinoa or brown rice

- Sliced avocado

- Shredded red cabbage

- Lime wedges

- Cilantro for garnish

Instructions:

- Arrange the roasted sweet potato cubes, cooked black beans, quinoa or brown rice, sliced avocado, and shredded red cabbage in a bowl.

- Garnish with lime wedges and cilantro.

- Drizzle with a simple lime vinaigrette made with lime juice, olive oil, salt, and pepper.

- **Tips for Crafting Nutrient-Packed Meals during Intermittent Fasting:**

Balanced Macronutrients:

Ensure your meals include a balance of protein, healthy fats, and complex carbohydrates to provide sustained energy.

Hydration is Key:

Stay hydrated during fasting periods. Water, herbal teas, and infused water with cucumber or mint are refreshing choices.

Portion Control:

Be mindful of portion sizes to prevent overeating during eating windows. Use smaller plates to create visually satisfying meals.

Whole Foods Emphasis:

Prioritize whole foods such as vegetables, fruits, lean proteins, and whole grains for optimal nutrient intake.

Experiment with Flavors:

Use herbs, spices, and citrus flavors to enhance the taste of your meals without relying on excessive salt or sugar.

Listen to Your Body:

Pay attention to hunger and fullness cues. If a particular eating window feels too restrictive, consider adjusting the fasting approach.

Customize to Preferences:

Tailor recipes to suit personal taste preferences and dietary restrictions. Flexibility is key to sustaining intermittent fasting.

Preparation is Key:

Plan your meals and prep ingredients in advance to streamline the cooking process, making it easier to stick to your fasting windows.

Incorporating these delicious and nutrient-packed recipes into your intermittent fasting routine can turn the eating windows into a culinary journey. By focusing on wholesome ingredients and mindful preparation, these meals not only align with the principles of intermittent fasting but also contribute to overall health and well-being. Remember to embrace variety, savor each bite, and enjoy the journey of nourishing your body in a way that feels both satisfying and sustainable.

THANKS FOR

READING

THIS BOOK.

www.ingramcontent.com/pod-product-compliance
Lightning Source LLC
Chambersburg PA
CBHW071052260726
48661CB00006B/2242